Yoga Bliss

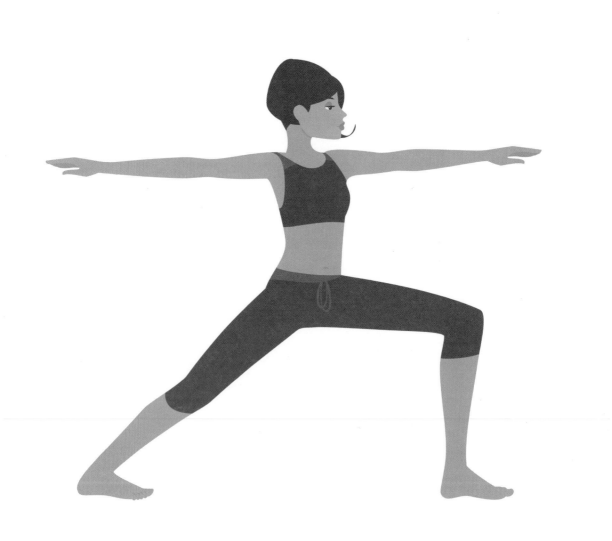

Yoga Bliss

simple and effective routines for chilling out

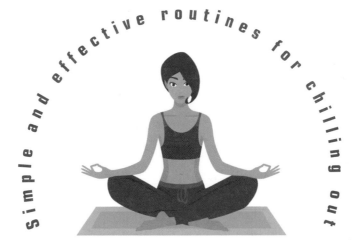

TARA FRASER

DUNCAN BAIRD PUBLISHERS

LONDON

Yoga Bliss
Tara Fraser

For Zoë, blissful baby.

First published in the United Kingdom and Ireland in 2007 by
Duncan Baird Publishers Ltd
Sixth Floor, Castle House
75-76 Wells Street
London W1T 3QH

Conceived, created and designed by Duncan Baird Publishers
Copyright © Duncan Baird Publishers 2007
Text copyright © Tara Fraser 2007
Commissioned artwork copyright © Duncan Baird Publishers 2007

The right of Tara Fraser to be identified as the Author of this text
has been asserted in accordance with the Copyright, Designs and
Patents Act of 1988.

All rights reserved. No part of this book may be reproduced in
any form or by any electronic or mechanical means, including
information storage and retrieval systems, without permission
in writing from the publisher, except by a reviewer who may
quote brief passages in a review.

Managing Editor: Grace Cheetham
Editors: Zoë Fargher and Kesta Desmond
Managing Designer: Daniel Sturges
Designer: Rachel Cross
Commissioned colour artwork: Roman Grey
Commissioned line artwork: Asami Mitsuhira for 3+Co.

British Library Cataloguing-in-Publication Data:
A catalogue record for this book is available from
the British Library

10 9 8 7 6 5 4 3 2

ISBN: 978-1-84483-383-2

Typeset in Eurostile and Trade Gothic
Colour reproduction by Colourscan, Singapore
Printed in China

Publisher's note:
Before following any advice or practice suggested in this book,
it is recommended that you consult a medical professional as to its
suitability, especially if you are pregnant, or suffer from any health
problems or special conditions. The publishers, the author and the
illustrators cannot accept responsibility for any injuries or damage
incurred as a result of following the exercises in this book, or of
using any of the therapeutic methods described or mentioned here.

Contents

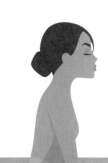

Introduction

Yoga is a wonderful antidote to the speed of modern living. It offers a practical method through which to reclaim genuine relaxation and ease. Practising yoga will alleviate built-up stress and tension, boost your energy, improve your health and, most importantly, make you feel better. Simple routines carried out with care for just a few minutes a day can transform your general outlook on your daily life. Some people devote their whole lives to these practices, but there is also a long and venerable tradition of the "householder yogi", an ordinary person who fits their practice around earning a living and sharing time and space with friends, family and colleagues, but who seeks to do this in a balanced, sustainable and beneficial way.

In this book I have included many postures that I regularly use myself and teach in my classes. They are not difficult or complicated, and people are often surprised how wonderful they feel afterwards. You may experience a whole range of benefits from even a basic practice, including better sleep, improved skin and hair, increased muscle tone, strength and flexibility, better mental health and feeling happier!

Yoga is not just exercise – it will equip you with the skills you need to help you live life to the full with a positive attitude and self-confidence. It is uniquely accessible and adaptable, and once begun, it can become a positive lifestyle habit – like brushing your teeth – and you may begin to wonder how you ever lived without your yoga! You do not need special equipment, a super flexible body, a perfectly calm environment or a great deal of spare time to practise yoga. A few minutes each day dedicated to these simple techniques, tried and tested by generations of busy people, can leave you feeling calmer, more alert and able to access deep reserves of energy within. Eventually, the release of tension and strain in your body and mind might just lead you back to the place that yoga says we all belong – the state of *ananda*, or bliss.

Chill out with yoga

Tranquillity, calm and stability are hard to find in our hectic modern world. Yoga originated in India thousands of years ago, and it is one of the most effective methods of bringing your mind and body back into balance, helping you to reach a longed-for state of "bliss".

This little book contains the basics of a home yoga practice, put together specifically to reduce stress or anxiety and to give you a sense of serenity and ease. The exercises are adaptations of classic yoga poses and should be fairly easy for anyone in generally good health. Some of these practices take just a few minutes to do – helping you to create a little oasis of calm every day.

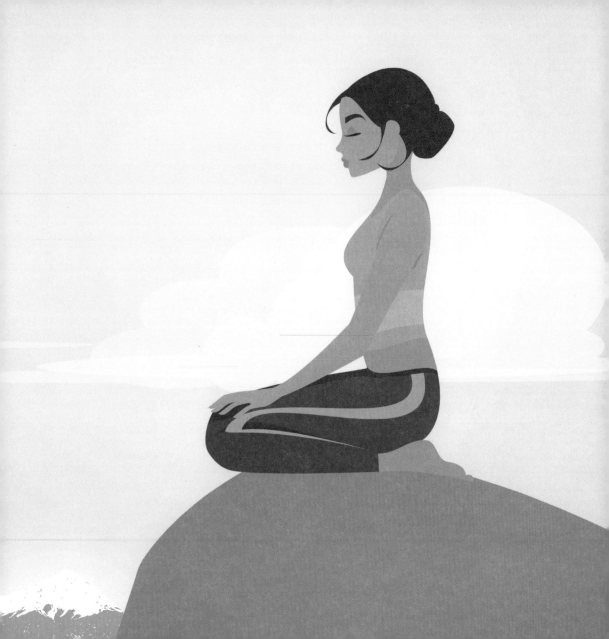

The path to bliss

According to the yoga tradition, our true nature is a state of *ananda* – bliss – and practising yoga will ultimately take us back toward this. Yoga takes a "whole person" approach to healing and restoring balance in our lives, accepting each person as an individual, with a unique constitution and life experience, so no two people will practise yoga in exactly the same way with exactly the same results. When you are practising, take into account not only your physical body, but also your mind, your emotions and the actions of your daily life. Being aware of all this, and its effects on you, will help to bring yourself back into a harmonious state of being.

It is important to realize that a yoga practice is not a fitness regime. You may find that you are more toned, supple and strong as a result of the exercises, but these physical benefits are not in themselves what you are working toward. You can be physically fit, but if you are also miserable or angry you are not in a state of yoga!

According to ancient yogic theory, we don't simply consist of a physical body plus a mind as we imagine in the West, but five *koshas* or bodies. These are:

1. *Annamaya-kosha*   ✦   **the physical body**
2. *Pranamaya-kosha*   ✦   **the energetic body (life-force)**
3. *Manomaya-kosha*   ✦   **the mental body**
4. *Vijnanamaya-kosha*   ✦   **the understanding body (or higher mind)**
5. *Anandamaya-kosha*   ✦   **the bliss body**

These five layers operate as a whole, explaining the phenomenon that if you are sick at heart, you'll become sick in mind or body too, and vice versa. Yoga encourages us to develop an awareness of ourselves in this multi-layered way. *Anandamaya-kosha* is perhaps easiest to overlook in our daily lives, but through awareness of it, you can connect to a place of great happiness, peace and repose. We all experience flashes of what it is to be connected fully with our "bliss body" – this book intends to show you how to get there by design rather than accident, through the process of yoga.

How to practise

Yoga works best if it is practised little and often, and this book is designed to help you achieve this. You can do these exercises on your own, or with a friend, in ordinary clothes, at home, or even in an office environment – so they're not exactly the same as the kind of thing you might do in a yoga class. The sequences are shorter and more focused than a long, athletic class with a teacher might be.

To get the most out of your yoga, it helps to have a few basic bits of equipment. A sticky yoga mat is useful, especially for standing postures as it gives your feet a nice secure grip. These are widely available in stores and online. You may find that a couple of foam yoga blocks come in handy too, although you could use a large book such as a telephone directory instead. If your knees are a bit fragile and you find kneeling poses uncomfortable, placing a folded blanket under them will give a little padding and protect your knee joints from injury.

Try to practise in a warm, well-ventilated space. Ideally, you should try to find somewhere free from clutter and distractions. In reality, most of us make do with the rooms we live in, which are both cluttered and full of distractions! At least turn off your cellphone, and choose a quiet time of day when you won't be disturbed.

Generally speaking, it's not a good idea to do yoga postures on a full stomach. Many people find that the ideal time to practise is first thing in the morning, before they have breakfast. However, this is not true of everyone, and both the sequences in Daily Routines would be fine to do an hour or so after a light meal – for example, you could do them in the evening after work.

Wear loose, comfortable clothes without restrictive belts or waistbands, and always practise barefoot. You can put some socks and perhaps an extra layer of clothing on at the end of your practice session, to keep your feet and body warm while you relax. If you wear contact lenses, you may prefer to take them out so that you can close your eyes comfortably for some of the exercises.

Basic principles

Yoga works on many different levels, and can ultimately provide you with the key to restoring balance, equilibrium and stability in your life. If you keep in mind a few basic principles, they will help to guide you toward a beneficial and enjoyable practice.

✦ Go slowly and carefully. We live in a high-speed age – everything around us is fast. Let your yoga be slow, gentle and deliberate. You are not in a hurry to achieve anything here, just take your time and be "in the moment".

✦ Yoga is not a competitive sport. These exercises are not designed to push you to some kind of athletic endurance threshold! Try not to compare yourself to other people or to how you were five or 10 years ago. Practising yoga is about how you are now, this moment, and working with the material you have. If you feel stiff, tired, tense and stressed then yoga can help you, but the first thing you must do is acknowledge those feelings and let them subside via your practice. Don't worry if some of these postures seem difficult to do at first – that's completely normal. You'll soon find that you'll get used to the new sensations.

✦ Work within your own limits. You won't progress more quickly by putting yourself through pain. Your body's natural response to pain is to tighten up and retract from it, making you feel worse, not better! In every exercise ensure that you feel no more than a moderate stretch. If you find yourself wincing, holding your breath or forcing yourself into postures, you have gone too far. Come back to your comfort zone and relax as fully as you can into the pose.

✦ Little and often. Yoga works best if you can do a little bit every day rather than a big long session once a week. If you consider all the little stresses that can build up daily, it makes sense to release them as they occur rather than allowing them to multiply until you feel frantic! A three-minute yoga practice is better than none at all; you just need to make a tiny space for it in your life, and it will soon become an easy and pleasurable habit.

✦ Breath is the essence of yoga. As you use the postures in this book, try to stay aware of the quality and speed of your breathing – it will give you a vital clue as to the quality of your performance of the postures. Our minds naturally tend to focus on the physical action rather than the breathing, so you will need to remind yourself of this time and time again.

You'll find that these basic principles will help you start and maintain your own yoga practice, so come back to them whenever you need to. You're ready to begin!

Three-minute stress busters

The techniques in this chapter can transform the way you feel in a matter of minutes. And the beauty of them is that they are easy to practise. You don't need lots of skill, experience or dedication!

Allowing yourself just a little time and space for these techniques can make the difference between feeling really dreadful and being able to cope. A situation that at first seemed impossible might feel more manageable after a few minutes of de-stressing. Practise one or more of these exercises whenever you feel life is getting too much – you may find you make better decisions, or deal with people in a more even-handed way.

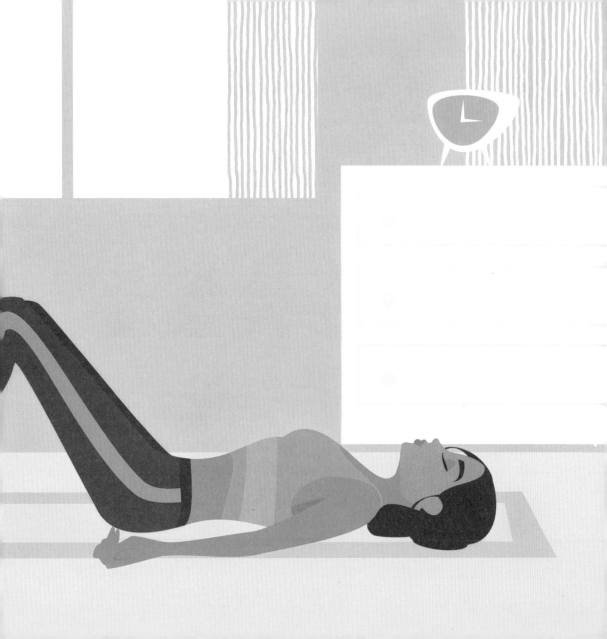

Semi-supine

This is an amazingly refreshing and relaxing posture. It's as easy as it looks and you can do it at any time. All you need is a bit of privacy and some floor space. You can stay in the semi-supine posture as long as you like, but three minutes is probably the minimum time you need to settle completely and begin to relax.

The semi-supine posture releases tension in your lower back and the area of your sacrum (the triangular bone at the base of your spine). Lying in a semi-supine position allows your spine and head to settle. The posture also eases anxiety, and releases tension stored in your upper back, neck and shoulders. Your breathing improves as your ribcage relaxes and your diaphragm has a little more freedom. You need to lie on the floor for this posture to work well – if you lie on a bed, the mattress doesn't give your body enough support.

✦ Lie on your back with your knees bent and your feet flat on the floor, about hip-width apart or slightly more. Let your knees fall in toward each other, or just leave them parallel. Rest your arms on the floor by your sides, palms up, a little way away from your body. If you like, you can rest your hands palm down on your lower abdomen, where you can feel the gentle movement of your breath.

Your head and neck should feel comfortable and your face should be parallel with the floor. If you feel your chin is tilting upward – or even if you don't – try putting a small cushion, slim paperback book or thin foam yoga block under your head to lift it a little. Close your eyes. Rest and breathe. Allow both your body and mind to be still and quiet for a few minutes.

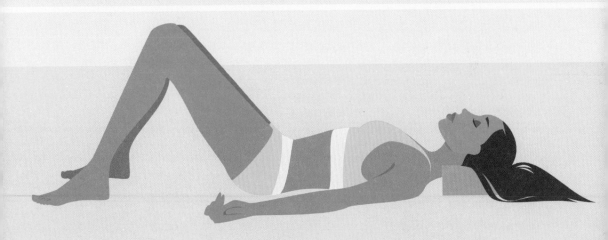

Figurehead

This pose is a fantastic way to stretch open your shoulders and the front of your chest. It counteracts the hunched-forward position that most of us tend to sit in at our computers or desks. When you do the pose, be aware that a little stretch goes a long way. You're not aiming to wrench your shoulders – you just want to achieve a soft, steady stretch that will gently open up your whole chest and shoulder area.

According to the theory of yoga, this pose stimulates the opening of the heart and throat chakras, which are responsible for unconditional love and communication – two things that we really need more of in most offices!

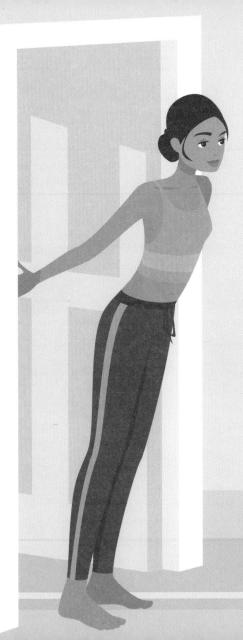

◆ Stand in a doorway and place your hands a little below shoulder level on the door frame. Walk forward until you can straighten your arms (raise or lower your hands so that you're comfortable). Stay like this for one or two minutes, breathing softly and evenly. As you inhale, feel the stretch flow to the centre of your chest and expand your heart; as you exhale, let your shoulders soften and open a little further. If the door frame is too narrow to do this pose, you can get the same benefits by holding a belt in both hands and gently swinging your arms up and behind you.

Ujjayi - take control

Ujjayi means "victorious" and its effect is exactly that – it lets you take control of your breathing and, as a result, your mind and emotions too. This technique simply involves slowing your breathing so that it becomes fuller and more even. This has an instantly de-stressing effect on your heart rate and nervous system, leaving you feeling relaxed yet alert. You can use *ujjayi* breath to keep you calm and focused in all sorts of challenging situations. It works well when you're walking at a steady pace or when you're sitting quietly.

Ujjayi breathing should not require great effort – it should feel easy and soft, and produce a relaxing and invigorating effect. Don't force your breath or let it become harsh or loud. It should just make a gentle hissing sound, pleasant to listen to.

Sit cross-legged or in any other comfortable position. Drop your chin slightly and join your thumbs and fingers in *chin mudra* (see pages 112–113). Lightly close the muscles in your throat so that you make a gentle hissing sound as you breathe out through your nose. Make the same hissing sound as you breathe in through your nose – you'll be using muscles higher up in your throat to do this. Keep the sound soft and even. Take 12 breaths or more in this way. You can increase the relaxing effect by making your out-breath up to twice as long as your in-breath. The reward is a relaxed and attentive mind.

Daily routines

Here are two yoga sequences to help you release mental and physical tension and restore a feeling of balance and serenity. They should take about 15 to 20 minutes each to complete and are made up of simple postures that are easy to learn and memorize.

The first sequence builds strength and uses more vigorous movements to help stimulate your body and free your mind of built-up stresses. The second allows time for staying in each pose to deepen the stretch and promote tranquillity. Try to practise one of these sequences daily – choose between them to suit your mood and the time of day, or combine them to make a longer practice.

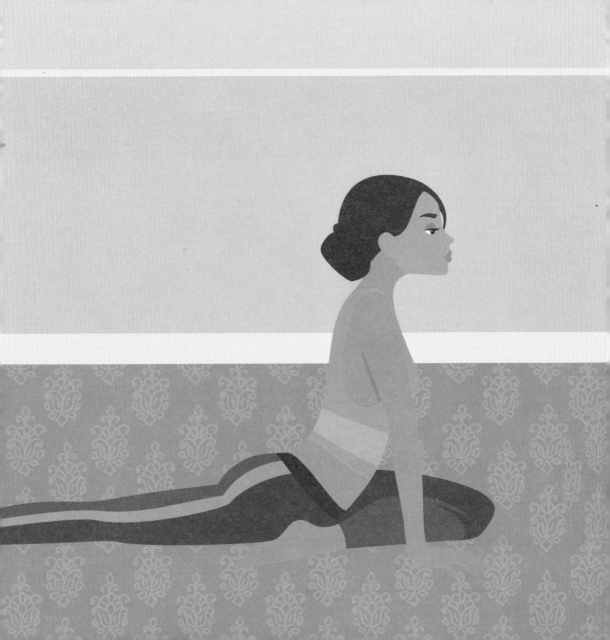

Forward bend

FIRST SEQUENCE

Forward bends are calming for your mind, and they quieten your nervous system. A deep forward bend creates a stretch that reaches from the back of your neck all the way down to the backs of your ankles. This opens the entire back surface of your body, allowing it to become softer and more flexible.

Simply bending forward is one of the most natural movements for the human body, but our modern lifestyles mean that many of us lose the ability to do this easily during childhood – and, often, never regain it! At first, you may feel alarmingly stiff when you attempt to bend forward, but you will improve rapidly over time as your muscles and joints start to free up. Treat your body very gently – your aim is to relax forward and release tension as you go, not to touch your toes!

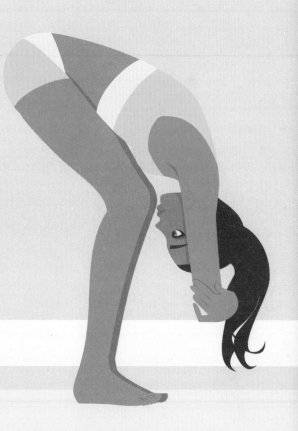

✦ Stand with your feet hip-width apart and parallel. Breathing in deeply, raise your arms over your head and stretch upward. As you breathe out, fold forward at your hips, and let your arms hang down toward the floor. Bend your knees a little to take the pressure off the backs of your legs. Make sure your knees are directly over your toes and that they don't "knock" or collapse toward each other.

To help relax your upper body, hold on to your elbows with your hands. This adds "weight" to your upper body so you can hang forward easily from your hips. Breathe deeply and steadily. To come up, gently release your arms and slowly uncurl your spine. Repeat this at least twice. Try to stay a little longer in the pose each time.

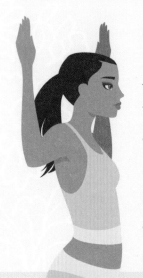

Warrior pose

This variation of a classical warrior posture will leave you feeling positive and uplifted. It improves the depth and strength of your in-breath, and encourages your chest and shoulders to open and expand. Position your arms carefully – don't push your elbows back beyond your shoulders as this can cause tension in your upper chest. This pose stimulates a powerful energy centre located in the middle of your chest (the *anahata chakra*).

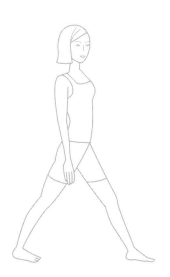

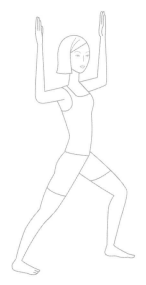

1 Step your left foot forward in a wide stride. Keep your hips facing forward. Breathing out, relax the back of your body. Root your back heel deeply into the floor. Lengthen up through your spine, drawing the crown of your head upward and dropping your tailbone downward so that there's a two-way stretch throughout your body.

2 Breathing in, bend your left knee and lift your arms to shoulder height, palms facing forward and elbows bent at right angles.

Repeat steps 1 and 2 at least six times with your left leg forward, and the same number of times with your right leg forward.

Cat pose

Keeping your spine strong and supple is essential for good health and all-round well-being. This simple pose will develop the flexibility of your spine. It will also increase your awareness of the muscles that support your back – particularly in the area of your lower abdomen. The key is not to rush. Maintain a calm focus on your body throughout the pose. Don't aim to achieve the end position as quickly as you can.

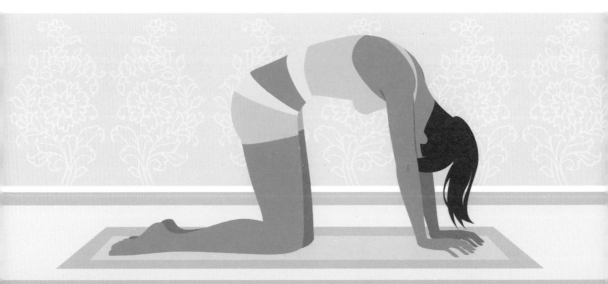

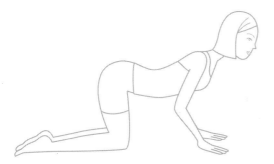 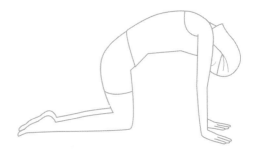

1 Position yourself on all fours and move your hands a little further forward than your shoulders. As you breathe in, bend your elbows slightly, drawing them back toward your knees. Lift and open the centre of your chest, sliding your shoulders down toward your waist and slightly raising your eye line. Keep your neck and throat muscles soft. Avoid pushing your chin forward or flinging your head back.

2 As you breathe out, gently release your head forward and drop your tailbone toward the floor until your back is fully rounded. Relax your shoulders so that they're not hunched around your neck. People tend to use their upper spine more in this position, but try to engage your abdominal muscles a little as well. This helps to focus your attention on deeply curving and rounding your lower back.

Repeat steps 1 and 2 at least six times – more if you can and if you're feeling the benefits. Let your movements flow into one another.

Down-facing dog

This refreshing, strengthening posture will invigorate your body and mind. It helps to build upper body strength, and stability in the core of your body. It also gives you a strong stretch in the backs of your legs. Down-facing dog is a very powerful pose and, even if you're quite fit, you may feel exhausted by your first few attempts. Keep practising, because it will become easier and easier and, eventually, you'll be able to sustain it for a long time! Gradually build up the length of time you stay in the posture, until you're able to hold it for a count of 12 breaths. Keep your breath smooth, soft and slow.

★ From an all-fours position, place your hands a little way in front of your shoulders, shoulder-width apart. Point your fingers straight forward and splay them out, opening your hands fully into the floor. Tuck your toes under, and push your hips up and back, lifting your sitting bones right up toward the ceiling.

Your arms should be straight, but if it's difficult to straighten your legs, bend your knees a little to take some of the pressure off. Your aim is to let your spine "hang" loosely from your hips, with your head relaxed between your elbows, and your shoulders wide and soft. Hold the pose for at least three breaths, then rest on all fours or in child pose (see pages 36–37) before repeating.

Pigeon pose

This graceful posture combines a deep, releasing stretch in your buttocks and the backs of your thighs with a steady, well-supported backbend. Move smoothly and gently from step to step, allowing your back to adjust to the pose little by little. This pose produces a powerful opening of your chest and throat area that can lift your spirits as well as release tension and stress.

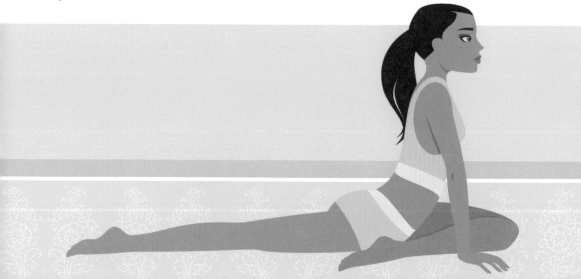

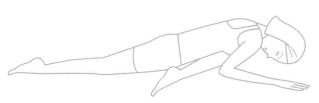

1 From an all-fours position, bring your left knee forward and take your left foot across your body, toward or, if possible, beyond your right hip. Lower your torso and head toward the floor. Stay here for at least four deep, steady breaths.

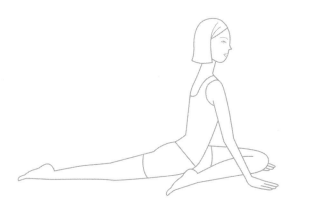

2 Place your hands just below your shoulders. As you breathe in, lift yourself into a gentle backbend. When you have gone as far as you can, breathe out and let the back of your body relax and your chest rise up a little more (if you feel pain in your back, lower yourself forward). Take four more breaths and gently release the pose. Repeat on the other side.

Child pose

This pose is simple, gentle and nurturing. It provides a wonderful antidote to stress and tension, and acts as a blissful release after almost any backbend. Bringing your head into contact with the earth often produces the sensation of allowing built-up tension to drain away, leaving you with a more relaxed and open perspective. You can relax in child pose for as long as you feel comfortable. If you don't find it easy at first, use a prop or change the position of your arms or legs as described opposite. There's no virtue in being uncomfortable in child pose – it's better to experiment until you feel relaxed. That way you can let your body and mind go completely.

⬧ Come into a kneeling position with your ankles and knees together. Lower your body forward until your head rests on the floor (or rest it on a thick book or yoga block).

Let your arms relax alongside your body with your hands resting palms up near your ankles. Alternatively, if it's more comfortable, rest your hands, palms down, on the floor close to your head.

Other ways to make this pose more comfortable include using a folded blanket as a padded surface, and opening your knees so that your chest rests in between them.

Stay in child pose for at least six breaths. Concentrate on relaxing your head, neck and shoulders and letting any strain or stress drain away from your head into the floor.

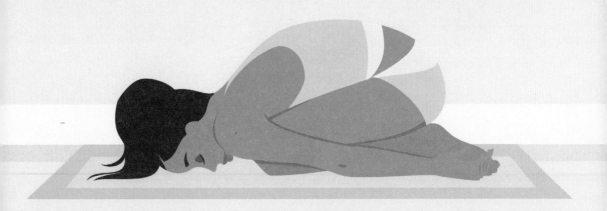

Squat

Using this posture for just a few minutes every day can be very beneficial for your whole body. Squatting is a basic, natural posture for the human body but, owing to the fact that we sit on chairs for much of our daily lives, most of us find it difficult at first. Regular practice of this posture will help to maintain and increase the health and flexibility of your spine, and keep your knees, hips and ankle joints supple and strong. Take care to align your knees, hips and ankles so that they're not under strain. This posture is also is good for your digestion and internal organs, and, because squatting requires you to balance, it will help you to focus and keep you mentally centred.

✦ Move from a standing position into a deep squat with your knees and feet turned out. Rest your elbows inside your knees and bring your hands together in front of your chest. If this is difficult, give yourself some help by placing a couple of books or yoga blocks underneath your heels. You can also practise this pose with your feet and knees parallel rather than turned out, and with your arms touching the floor in front of you to help you balance. Find the variation of the pose that's most comfortable for you.

When you're in the pose, try gently rocking forward and backward or side to side – this makes the pose less strenuous for your muscles and can help you to relax into the pose for longer. When you need to, gently drop your head forward, lift your hips and roll up your spine to come back to standing.

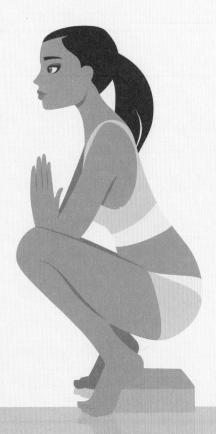

Knees-to-chest pose

**SECOND
SEQUENCE**

The traditional Sanskrit name for this posture is *apanasana*, which means "the posture of the downward force of energy". *Apana* energy cleanses and purifies both your body and mind. This pose gently stimulates the muscles and connective tissue around your sacrum (the triangular bone at the base of your spine) and lower back, parts of the body that are often under huge strain in daily life.

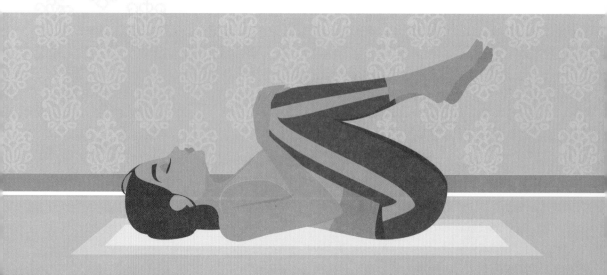

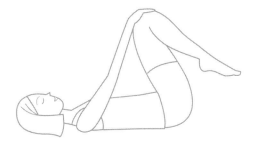

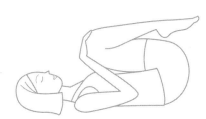

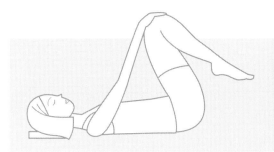

1 Lie on your back. Breathing out, draw your knees toward your chest. Rest one hand on the top of each knee, fingers pointing to your toes. This keeps your upper body soft and relaxed, especially around your shoulders.

2 As you inhale, allow your knees to roll gently away from your chest until your arms are straight. This movement may be small, but you should feel a gentle release through the whole of your lower spine and sacrum.

* If you feel your chin is sticking up in the air in this pose, use a slim book or a yoga block under your head to add a little support. This will keep the back of your neck long and relaxed.

Stirrup pose

This simple but effective exercise will increase the mobility in your hips and give you a sense of ease and freedom in the whole of your lower back, hip and sacrum area. It's the same movement that we all did as tiny babies, holding onto our toes – rediscover your inner child! Practise this posture regularly to reduce strain on your spine, and to help prevent lower back pain.

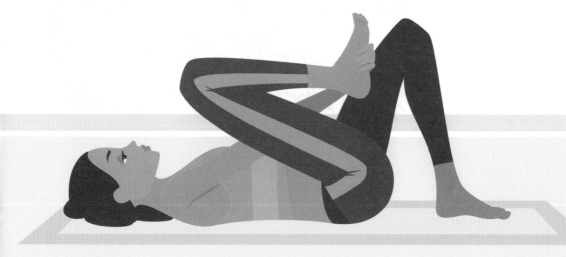

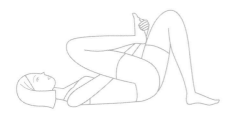
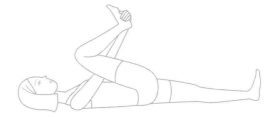

1 From knees-to-chest pose (see pages 40–41), bring your right hand to the inside of your right leg and hold your right instep. Let your left foot settle on the floor with your left knee bent, and relax your left arm by your side. Let your right shoulder release as you move your right leg in small circles to the left and right. Do this for at least eight breaths.

2 If it's possible – and comfortable – very gently and slowly relax your left leg right down to the floor. This will produce a much stronger stretch in your hips and legs. Focus your mind on the movement you make in your hip sockets, relaxing and opening the joint all the time. Keep the posture soft and mobile. Repeat on the other side.

* Many people experience strain in their shoulders and the back of the neck when they first try this posture. Move slowly and gently, and place a block or book under your head to reduce strain if you need to. Allow your head to stay heavy and relaxed.

Bridge pose

After the stirrup pose (see pages 42–43), this pose opens your hip sockets in the other direction. Bridge pose is a gentle backbend that will enhance your breathing capacity, give you a flexible spine and strong legs, and help your shoulders and neck to relax. If you used a book or a yoga block under your head for the last posture, remove it for this one.

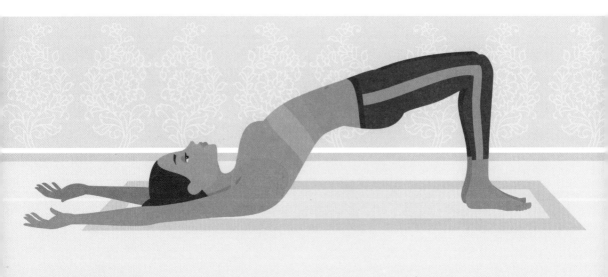

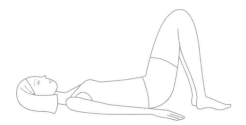

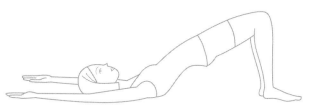

1 Lie on your back and place both feet firmly on the floor, about hip-width apart, with your knees bent and parallel. Relax your arms on the floor by your sides and breathe out.

2 As you breathe in, push into the floor firmly with both feet and lift your hips gently upward as far as is comfortable. At the same time raise your arms over your head. Repeat the whole exercise four to eight times.

* To allow the entire back surfaces of your arms to rest on the floor in an easy way, you may need to let your arms swing open to a wide position. This will allow your neck and shoulders to relax too. Bend your elbows as much as you like.

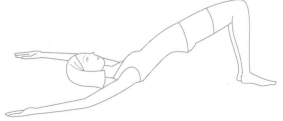

Reclining tailor pose

Reclining tailor pose is a wonderful posture for relaxation. It works as a restorative posture, where you can re-connect to your awareness of your breath, and settle your mind. This pose is also good for relieving tension and strain, and it helps your hips to become free and mobile.

When you're in the posture, let your shoulders and ribcage rest easily on the floor and allow your head and pelvis to become very heavy. Soften the muscles in your face, scalp and neck as you relax your shoulders and chest. Give yourself time to "melt" into the pose, so that your whole body can become deeply relaxed and open. When you come out of the pose, do so gently, drawing your knees together with the help of your hands and rocking gently on your back a few times.

Lie on your back, place the soles of your feet together and let your knees fall to the sides. Place your hands on your lower abdomen where you can feel the gentle movement of your breath. Hold the pose for at least eight breaths, or many more if you're comfortable.

You may need support from props to make this pose really relaxing. Try putting a yoga block or book under your head. Support your knees with a couple of big cushions or blocks – this will allow your hips to relax and open. If they're under strain, they can become tense.

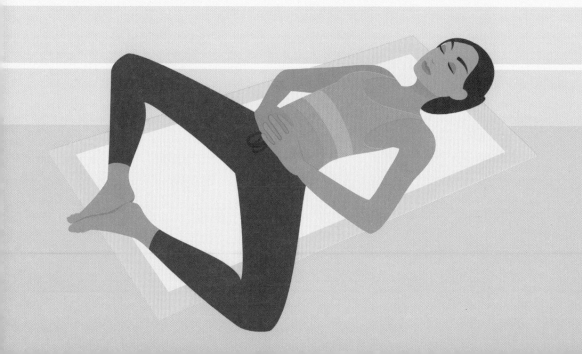

Spinal twist

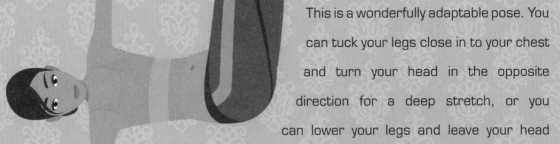

This is a wonderfully adaptable pose. You can tuck your legs close in to your chest and turn your head in the opposite direction for a deep stretch, or you can lower your legs and leave your head central for a softer, easier stretch. Either way, this pose stimulates your spinal nerves, keeps your spine mobile, and relieves tension in your whole body – making you feel blissfully relaxed.

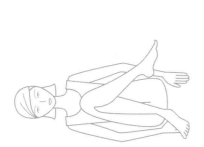

1 Lie on your back, tuck your knees in toward your chest and then cross your right leg over your left.

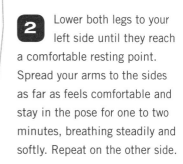

2 Lower both legs to your left side until they reach a comfortable resting point. Spread your arms to the sides as far as feels comfortable and stay in the pose for one to two minutes, breathing steadily and softly. Repeat on the other side.

* If you find it difficult to cross your legs in the pose, then try keeping your knees and ankles together instead. A small cushion or block under your head can make the pose more comfortable.

Leg raise

This simple leg-raising exercise is a fantastic way to synchronize your breath with your movement. This is a key aspect of yoga that, once mastered, can be a quick and practical method of changing your state of mind from anxious, tense or overloaded to cool and calm. Leg raises will also deepen your breathing, and work the muscles of your torso and your hips. Although this pose is simple, it requires mental concentration and abdominal strength!

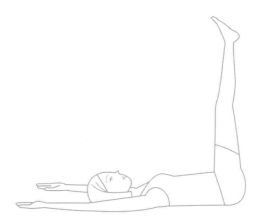

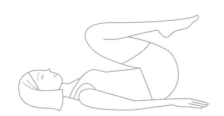

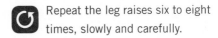

1 Lie on your back with your knees tucked in toward your chest and your arms resting beside you. If you feel more comfortable with a little bit of support under your head, add a book or yoga block to help relax your neck and shoulders. Breathe out.

2 As you breathe in, lift your arms over your head. Let them relax on the floor behind you. Simultaneously lift your legs until they're roughly straight. Breathe out to return to step 1. Repeat, allowing the movement of your arms, legs and breath to work perfectly together.

Repeat the leg raises six to eight times, slowly and carefully.

Resting pose

This classic resting posture appears in some very old yoga texts, alongside much more athletically demanding poses. This gives an indication of the importance of resting pose in providing a contrast to strong physical work. Although this posture is simple, it can be difficult to let yourself go if you're feeling tense and stressed. Nevertheless, the results of just attempting it can be beneficial.

Maintain a constant awareness of what you are doing in the posture – it's not the same as going to sleep! Ideally, you should be absolutely physically still and mentally quiet at the same time. Physical stillness is not too much of a problem: it's mental quiet that's the real challenge for most of us. With practice, however, you'll discover that this pose is wonderfully restful for both your body and mind.

◆ Lie on the floor on your back. Put a book or yoga block under your head if you like, and, unless it's very warm, cover yourself with a blanket or shawl. Your body temperature will drop while you are lying still.

Place your feet a little way apart, and allow your legs to relax completely. Relax your arms by your sides with your palms facing upward. Close your eyes.

Once you are settled comfortably, resist any urge to move again for the next few minutes. Breathe through your nose, letting your breath be smooth and calm. Make a mental note of when you're breathing in and when you're breathing out. Each time you catch yourself thinking of something else, take your mind back to observing your breath. Do this for at least 12 breaths, or much longer if you can.

Make sure you come out of the posture slowly and gently. To complete your practice, roll onto your right side, and push yourself up to sitting.

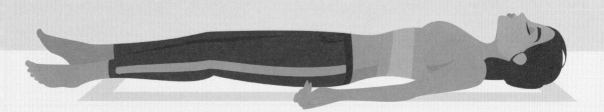

Weekend routine

This chapter contains a 16-posture sequence that's slightly more vigorous than the previous sequences. It's perfect for when you have a little more time – for example, at the weekend. The whole sequence should take 40 to 60 minutes. Some of the postures will be familiar to you by now. Try to memorize the sequence so you can focus on the postures rather than looking at the book.

Adding any of the breathing or meditation exercises in the following chapters to the end of this sequence will make a rounded yoga practice. A routine of this type will leave you refreshed and replenished, with increased mental energy and focus.

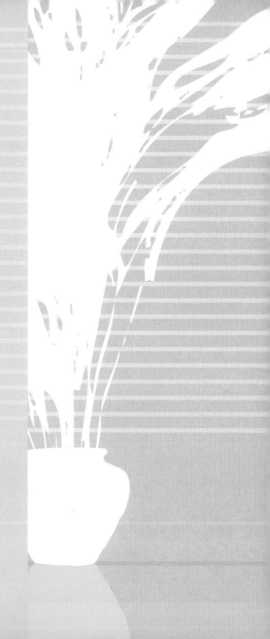

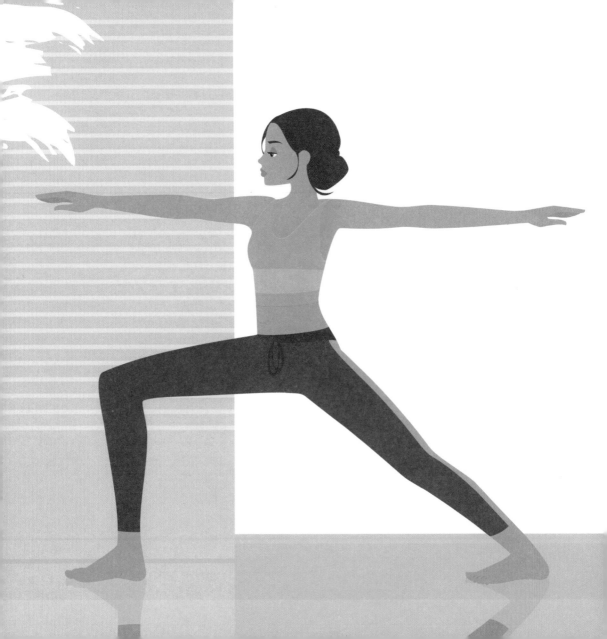

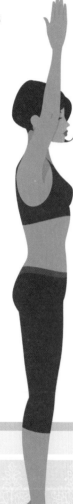

Upright stretch

Although this seems like a simple little exercise, you may need quite a bit of practice to master it. Your balance is linked to how you're feeling emotionally – if you can physically balance, you may find it easier to approach emotional concerns more calmly. This exercise will also develop your core strength, stability and co-ordination.

Make each part of your movement smooth and precise. You should be totally in control all the way through, with your movements synchronized perfectly with your breath.

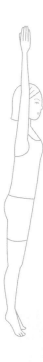

1 As you breathe in, gently raise your arms overhead. At the same time lift your heels until you're balancing on the balls of your feet and your toes. Allow your body to lengthen, extending the sides of your waist, and reaching up with your arms as far as you can.

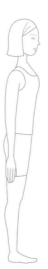

2 As you breathe out, make a controlled descent onto your heels and lower your arms back to your sides. The secret of this exercise is to synchronize the length of your breath with the tiny movement of your feet and the much bigger movement of your arms. You'll need to drop your heels very slowly.

Take your time and do at least six to eight calm, steady repetitions before moving on to the next pose.

Forward bend

This forward bend also appears in Daily Routines, but here the stretch is deeper – this will help you to develop flexibility in your legs. Intense stretching will also stimulate your body, and help release tension and stress. You may find this posture quite taxing in the backs of your legs, particularly in your hamstrings. Afterwards, however, you may well experience a sense of being fully relaxed and you may even enjoy a better night's sleep.

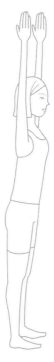

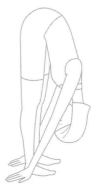

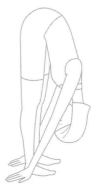 If the backs of your legs feel uncomfortable, and keeping them straight strains your lower back, try bending your knees a little.

1 Stand with your feet parallel and about hip-width apart. Make sure your knees are aligned directly over your toes and that they don't roll inward toward each other. Take a deep breath as you lift your arms overhead, stretching strongly upward.

2 As you breathe out, fold forward at your hips. Bring your fingertips to the floor behind your feet, or to your shins – wherever is comfortable. Allow the movement of your next in-breath to lengthen your spine. Stay in the pose for four to six breaths.

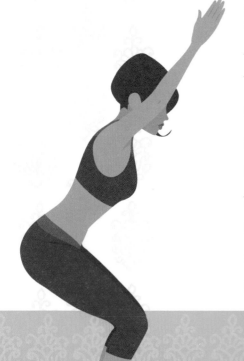

Standing squat

The traditional Sanskrit name for this posture is *utkatasana*, and it is sometimes called the "mighty pose". You should have a feeling of grounded, powerful strength while you practise it. Imagine that your body is thrusting upward from your hips, your waist is lengthening and your feet are deeply rooted in the ground. This pose helps to build strength in your legs and back.

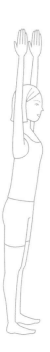

1 Stand with your feet approximately hip-width apart and parallel. As you breathe in, raise your arms above your head, keeping them about shoulder-width apart, with your palms facing in toward each other.

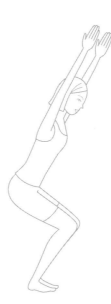

2 As you breathe out, bend your knees, making sure that they're directly over your toes so that your knees are nice and stable. Squat down as far as you can with your heels still in contact with the floor. Keep your head and neck in line with your spine. As you breathe in, straighten your knees again. Breathe out to lower your arms slowly back down by your sides.

Repeat steps 1 and 2 four to six times. Do more repetitions if the exercise feels comfortable. Keep your movements slow and careful.

Warrior pose

This posture will develop your stamina and strength, and leave you feeling positive and uplifted. It helps to increase flexibility in your hips and groin. You can practise the pose dynamically (moving in and out of the posture, inhaling and exhaling in time with your movements), or statically. Dynamic movements are a little easier.

Doing the pose statically demands more stamina and endurance. You can choose to work either way, depending on how you feel.

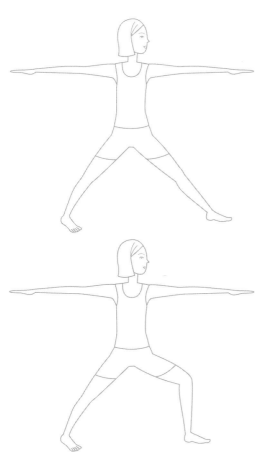

1 Place your feet wide apart. Turn your left foot out to 90 degrees and turn the toes of your right foot inward, so you have a good grip with your heel. As you breathe in, raise your arms to shoulder height, palms facing down. Turn your head to look along your left arm.

2 As you breathe out, bend your left knee deeply. Make sure that your left knee is directly above your left ankle. Your right hip should roll outward, so that you feel a stretch in your hip sockets, groin and abdomen. Maintain a vertical, warrior-like stance. Repeat the whole exercise with your right leg in front, looking along your right arm.

Asymmetrical forward bend

This pose will improve your balance and help you co-ordinate your breath with your movements. It's a great way to release tension in the back of your body and it gives your hamstrings a wonderful stretch. Relax your face, neck, shoulders and upper back muscles as you breathe out – these are often the first areas to get tense when you're stressed, and the last to relax.

1 Stand with your feet together. Step your left foot in front. Keep it parallel and pointing forward. Your right foot can turn out slightly if it's more comfortable. Try to keep your right heel in contact with the floor at all times. As you breathe in, slowly raise your arms above your head.

2 Breathing out, bend your front knee and fold forward. Bring your hands to the floor on either side of your left foot. Take two easy breaths. As you breathe in again, lift up to standing. Repeat three times, then repeat the whole exercise on the other side.

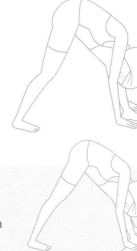

* If your hands don't reach the floor easily, it's fine to place a couple of yoga blocks or thick books under them so that you get the feeling of touching down to earth and releasing fully.

Tiger pose

This is a key posture for developing mindful awareness of your body. It's also important for developing flexibility in your spine and strength in your abdomen. Practise the movements slowly and gracefully to make the most of this simple but effective posture. Keep your chin and throat soft as you gently raise your head and extend your neck.

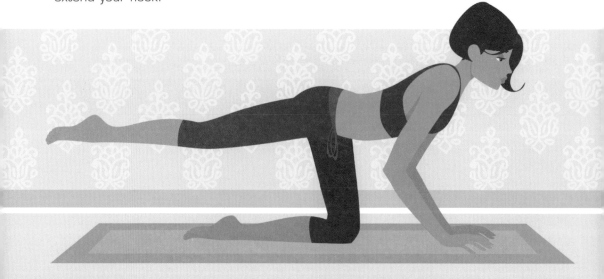

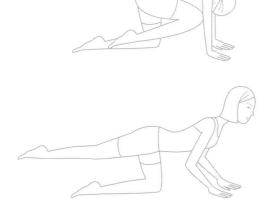

1 Begin in an all-fours position. As you breathe out, draw your right knee in toward your chest, tucking your head in and rounding your back as fully as you can – you may be able to touch your nose to your knee. Deeply draw in the muscles of your abdomen.

2 As you breathe in, stretch out your right leg behind you and slightly soften your elbows so they bend back (toward your knees, not out to the sides). Slip your shoulder blades back and down toward your waist as you allow your chest to open up and move forward between your arms.

↻ Repeat steps 1 and 2 at least four to six times with your right leg and then four to six times with your left leg. Move in a smooth, controlled way.

Down-facing dog

Down-facing dog is a fantastic posture for building strength and stamina. These qualities may not seem all that important when your main aim is to relax, but a degree of staying power and a solid foundation will restore your body's natural balance, allowing it to function efficiently. The effort you need to sustain the pose may also help to release pent-up stress and tension.

This posture is regarded as an "inversion" in yoga. Inverted postures are said to change the way energy circulates in the body and have a purifiying and calming effect. This is the same pose that you did in the first sequence of Daily Routines, but here you sustain the pose a little longer and more vigorously.

Kneel with your feet hip-width apart and place your hands on the floor, shoulder-width apart and parallel. Open your hands fully into the floor, letting your weight spread through your whole hand. Tuck your toes underneath you and lift your hips up and back. Extend your back, broaden your shoulders and lift your sitting bones toward the ceiling. Press your heels steadily to the floor, keeping your back and your legs straight. Let your head relax and keep your shoulders wide and soft. Hold the pose for at least four breaths, then rest on all fours and repeat. Work up to holding the pose for 12 breaths. If you feel discomfort in your wrists and shoulders, come out of the pose.

Swan pose

Like child pose (see pages 36–37), this relaxed posture will de-stress and soothe your lower back, restoring balance and harmony to your body and mind. Resting your head between your hands will encourage you to focus inwardly, steady your breathing after the exertion of the previous postures and help you to absorb the benefits of the sequence so far. You can also practise swan pose by itself when you want to get into a calm, relaxed frame of mind, or when your lower back is feeling strained and tense. Resting in this pose before you go to sleep at night can help you to unwind and let go of the tensions of the day.

From down-facing dog (see pages 68–69), relax your knees back down to the floor and sit back with your hips against your heels. Fold your hips, knees and ankles together completely, so you can rest your head on the floor. To relieve any pressure on your feet or ankles, place a rolled-up towel under your ankles. If your hips don't touch your heels, place a yoga block or a cushion under your hips, and if your head doesn't reach the floor, place a yoga block or a couple of books under your forehead. Gently extend your hands forward, palms facing down, and release your shoulders. Once you're comfortable, stay here for at least eight breaths, allowing your body to rest and relax.

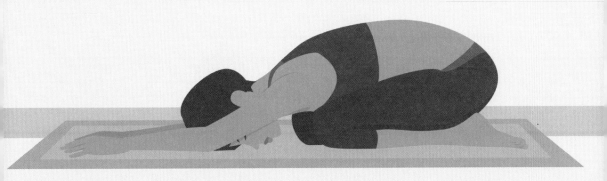

Hero pose

You can practise this powerful and steady pose to centre your energy and re-gather your strength. It will rest your legs, but also provide a steady stretch in your ankles. If you find hero pose easy, it's an ideal meditation posture. The key is to release your whole body downward, giving you a feeling of relaxation and serenity, but also of being securely grounded.

If you used some padding to help relax your knees or ankles in swan pose (see pages 70–71), leave it in place for this posture too, or sit on a block. If you feel any discomfort, come out of the posture and try it again using some more padding. It's worth taking the time to get the padding just right, to allow you to relax completely.

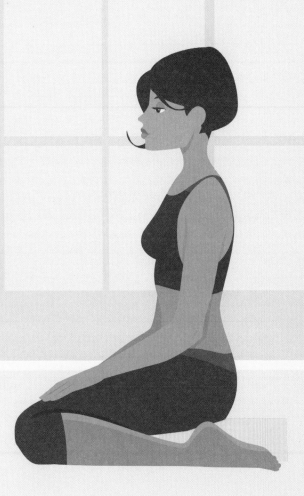

◆ Come up to a kneeling position. Rest your hands on your thighs, palms facing down, and release your weight down into your hips and then through your hips toward the floor. Release your lower back so that your pelvis is perfectly vertical and your spine is strong and upright.

Allow your shoulders to relax downward, while keeping your collar bones broad and open. Let your head balance easily on your neck, and tuck in your chin fractionally. This will encourage the back of your neck to stay long and open.

Try to remain totally still and to be aware of your breathing. Take six steady, soft breaths in this position and then move on to the next pose.

Frog pose

This is a deeply relaxing posture. It's a variation of swan pose (see pages 70–71), which will leave you feeling centred, balanced and released. Like swan pose, frog pose involves a really deep fold in your hips, knees and ankles. However, because your knees are wide apart, the angle of your back changes, and you may find that you're able to make almost a concave shape with your spine. This makes the pose a combination of a calming forward bend at your hips and an energizing backbend in your spine. As in swan pose, you may need to put a block between your hips and heels, or a rolled-up towel under your ankles to make this exercise really comfortable. Taking long, deep breaths in this pose will add to its calming, centring effect.

★ From the previous pose, spread your knees so they're wide apart. Keep your toes pointing toward each other and nearly touching. Fold forward and lower yourself to the ground, making sure your buttocks remain in contact with your heels. You can support yourself with your elbows and hang your head forward or, if possible, drop lower still so that you're able to rest your head on your forearms or the floor.

If you're very flexible, you'll find that you can relax your chest to the floor in this pose. If so, turn your head to one side for a few breaths and then to the other for a few more. See if you can stay here for at least eight breaths – rest for many more if you're comfortable. Gently push yourself back up and lie down on your back ready for the next pose.

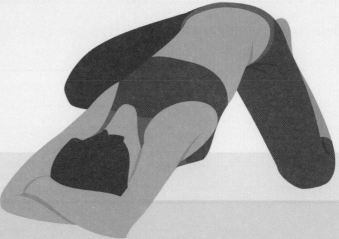

Twist

According to the theory of yoga, twisting postures purify the body because they stimulate our internal systems and organs to cleanse themselves. Twisting will remove any feeling of sluggishness and help you to feel brighter and more alert. Mentally and emotionally, a deep twist like this one may help you to move out of a rut or take a different perspective on a situation. Quite apart from all of this, twisting helps to build flexibility and strength in your spinal column. It also makes you more aware of your breath and develops your breathing capacity – all round, this is a very important pose!

Lie on your back and spread your arms out to the sides roughly in line with your shoulders. Let them relax. Draw your knees toward your chest. As you breathe out, gently lower your knees to the right side of your body, allowing your right knee to touch the floor. Rest your legs completely. If your knees don't reach the floor easily, you can prop them up with a cushion or a yoga block to make the pose more comfortable.

Gently turn your head to look over your left shoulder. Keep your neck soft and relaxed. Stay in this position for at least six breaths on each side, more if you can. A variation of this pose is to cross your legs before you twist. If you cross your right leg over your left, twist to the left and vice versa.

Bridge pose

This gentle backbend helps to open your chest, enabling you to breathe more fully. It also releases your shoulders, which can become hunched and tight in the stresses and strains of daily life. Bridge pose creates strength and stability in your pelvic floor, and legs and lower abdomen. Make sure that you continue to breathe evenly and smoothly throughout the movements, so that you feel no sense of strain.

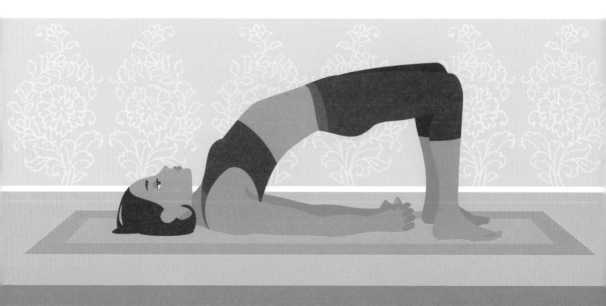

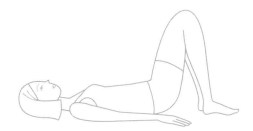

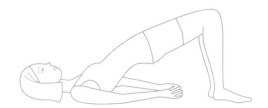

1 Lie on your back with your knees bent and your feet planted firmly on the floor, hip-width apart. Check that your feet are parallel – it's easy for them to turn out slightly at the toes. Place your hands on the floor beside your hips with your palms facing down.

2 As you breathe in, press your feet and hands firmly into the floor. You'll feel your hips lift – take them as far up as you can without straining. Clasp your hands behind your back, and push your knuckles toward your heels. Rock slightly from side to side in order to get your shoulder blades tucked right in beneath you. Hold the pose for three to six breaths, then come down gently. Repeat two or three times.

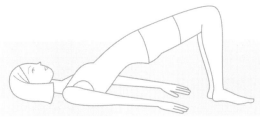

* If your shoulders feel uncomfortable when you clasp your hands in this pose, place your palms flat on the floor.

Unsupported shoulderstand

Inverted yoga postures, such as shoulderstand, calm your mind and can encourage restful sleep. In a classic shoulderstand, you use your hands and arms to support your body. In this variation your arms are stretched beyond your head and you use your abdominal muscles to support yourself instead. The arm position reduces the pressure on your neck and shoulder area.

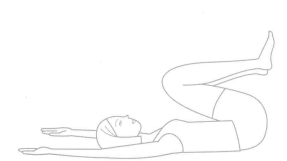

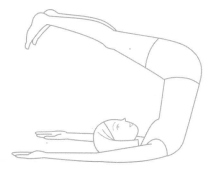

1 Lie on your back and gently hug your knees toward your chest. Leave your knees tucked in and raise your arms over your head. Rest the whole length of your arms on the floor – to do this you may need to bend your elbows and widen the space between your arms. Let all the tension go from your arms, shoulders, neck and throat. If you want to continue into shoulderstand, you can, but it's also fine to rest in this position and concentrate on your breath.

2 As you breathe out, leave your arms heavy on the floor behind you and contract your abdominal muscles to help you swing your legs overhead and lift your hips off the floor. If you find this difficult, use your hands to push into the floor beside your hips. Move into a semi-upright position. The higher you lift your legs, the more abdominal strength you'll need. Hold this position for four to 10 breaths and then carefully roll back down to the floor and relax.

Boat pose

Boat is a seated balance posture that demands clear mental focus and a strong torso. It's a demanding posture, but you can hold it for a short time at first and then gradually work up to holding it for longer. Take care – as with all yoga poses – that the effort of the posture doesn't create tension around your face and neck. Keep your jaw soft, your tongue relaxed and your eyes steady as you hold the pose.

Boat pose will improve your overall posture and core strength, but ensure that you're balancing on your sitting bones with a straight spine – this is not a stomach crunch! If you feel as if you're rounding your back, or if you have a tendency to roll over backward, bring your legs a little lower to start with, and focus on lifting and opening your chest.

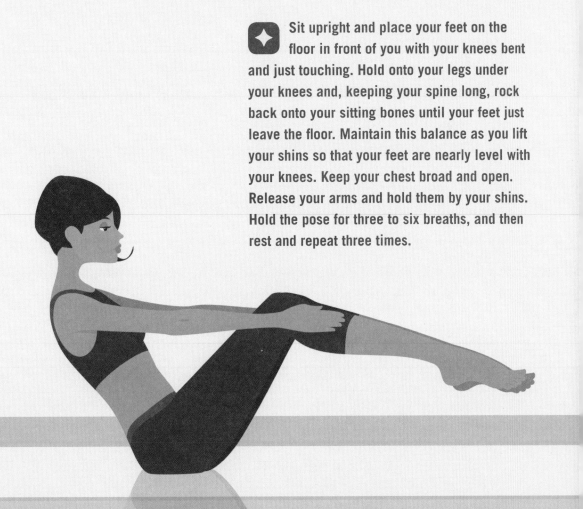

✦ Sit upright and place your feet on the floor in front of you with your knees bent and just touching. Hold onto your legs under your knees and, keeping your spine long, rock back onto your sitting bones until your feet just leave the floor. Maintain this balance as you lift your shins so that your feet are nearly level with your knees. Keep your chest broad and open. Release your arms and hold them by your shins. Hold the pose for three to six breaths, and then rest and repeat three times.

Tailor pose

This posture opens your hips and encourages them to relax outward, allowing your spine to rise effortlessly upward from the base of your pelvis. It's a basic sitting position and the human body is well adapted to it – once they can sit up, babies naturally adopt this position. Having said this, you may find tailor pose surprisingly difficult unless you already spend a lot of your time sitting on the floor. The use of furniture such as chairs and sofas from an early age means that most adults in the West are just not used to getting into a position like this. You could try using this position in daily life, as well as part of your yoga routine. Rather than sitting on the sofa to watch television, try sitting in tailor pose on the floor or on a cushion – as with all yoga postures, practise little and often and you'll soon make progress.

⬥ Sit on the floor and bring the soles of your feet together. Let your knees drop to the sides in a relaxed way. Ideally, your spine should be perfectly straight, so if your back is rounded and your knees are up near your shoulders, add a yoga block or a couple of thick books under your hips to raise the level of your pelvis a bit. If you feel a strong stretch in your inner thighs, you can prop your knees up with cushions or blocks to relieve the pressure. Hold onto your shins and lengthen your spine as you breathe in. As you breathe out, let your hips and knees become heavy and relaxed. Stay for six to 12 breaths, and then relax in the next posture.

Resting pose

Although you may be tempted to skip this final pose and move on to the next thing in your day, don't! At the end of a yoga sequence it's really important to take some time to allow your whole body to release completely. Resting pose creates a vital balance in your practice. Without it, you'll have stimulated your physical body and energetic system and left it buzzing. This creates an imbalance – it might feel good for a while, but you'll feel exhausted later on.

There is an idea in yoga that you need a period of absorption or digestion after practising postures. During this time, the work you've done filters through your various layers of being until it becomes a part of you. If you don't relax at the end of a yoga practice, you risk leaving your work "undigested", so that it's never fully absorbed, and is less effective as a result.

★ Lie on the floor with a little support under your head if you like. Cover yourself with a blanket or shawl unless it's very warm – your body temperature will drop while you are lying still.

Let your feet rest a little way apart and allow your legs to relax completely. Relax your arms at your sides with your palms facing up. Close your eyes and let the muscles of your face and head release and become soft and smooth. Become aware of your breath and allow it to be soft and natural. It can be helpful to keep your attention gently focused on the sensation of breath in one physical place, perhaps at the edge of your nostrils, the bridge of your nose or the back of your throat. Each time you catch yourself thinking of something else, bring your mind gently back to your breath. Stay for at least 12 breaths, or longer if you can. Don't fall asleep!

Take care to come out of the posture slowly and gently. Roll to your right side and push yourself up to a sitting position to complete your practice.

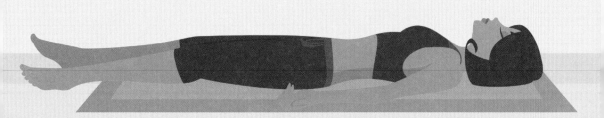

Breathe easy

The speed, depth and quality of your breathing reflects not only how hard you're exercising, but also your mental and emotional state. If you're tense and stressed, your breathing pattern will typically become shorter, with your breath held higher in your chest area.

The exercises in this chapter will develop, lengthen and deepen your breath so that it's full, easy and slow, helping you to achieve a relaxed mental state. You can practise these simple techniques on their own, or combine them with postures to create a longer routine, perhaps at the weekend. Don't do all these breathing practices one after the other – just select one at a time and concentrate on that.

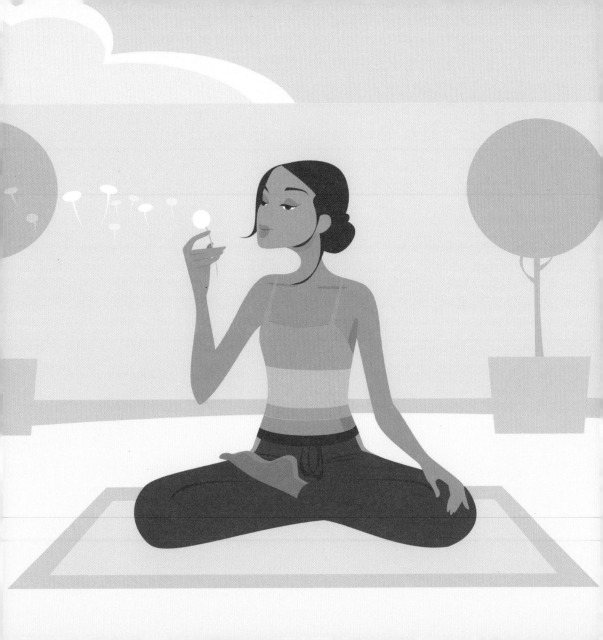

Sshhh - quietening breath

When you learn new breathing patterns in yoga, your first priority is to lengthen your out-breath. This helps your body and mind to relax and unwind. In this exercise you use a vocalized "sshhh" sound so you can hear how fast you're breathing, and use this sound to slow down your breath. You may be able to double the length of your out-breath over time using this exercise. Let your movements be small and easy.

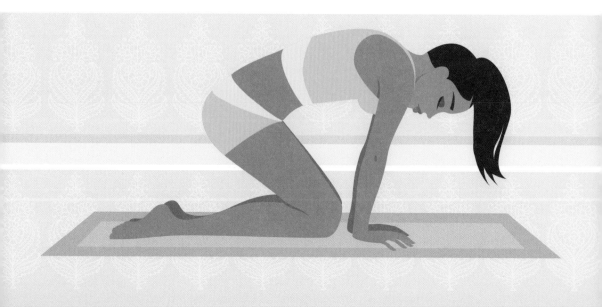

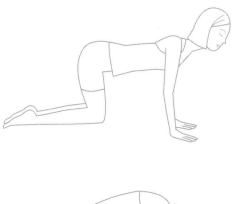

1 On your hands and knees, make a gentle version of the cat pose on pages 30–31. As you breathe in, gently let your chest open. Allow your elbows to bend a little to help you keep your shoulders soft, and let your back bend so that it's slightly concave.

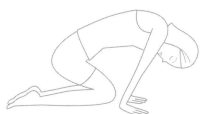

2 As you exhale, let your breath come out through your mouth and make a "sshhh" sound. At the same time, draw your lower abdomen in softly, and let your head curl in toward your tailbone. Keep moving only as long as you can make the sshhh sound – when you run out of breath, allow yourself to breathe in gently and come back to step 1.

↺ Repeat the whole exercise six to eight times, each time allowing your out-breath to be as complete as possible without forcing it.

Ujjayi - victorious breath

The basic method for this breathing technique is explained on pages 22–23. *Ujjayi* breath involves slightly restricting the amount of air that travels through your throat as you breathe. The effect of this is to slow down both your inhalation and your exhalation. You should practise *ujjayi* breath extremely gently and softly. As with several other yoga breathing exercises, this technique uses the slight hissing sound of the air passing through your throat to help keep your attention continuously on your breath. This way you know immediately when your breath is starting to lose its soft quality and become forced or strained.

Breathe in and out using the *ujjayi* technique. Make your in-breath exactly the same length as your out-breath. To do this accurately you'll need to count both in your head. Do at least eight breaths to make sure you can keep the ratio consistent and don't have to add a little catch-up breath somewhere in between. Now try changing the ratio of the length of your out-breath compared to your in-breath. Gradually lengthen your out-breath a count at a time until it's up to twice the length of your in-breath. This is a very pacifying and calming pattern, which may take you some weeks of practice to achieve. You'll notice that on days when you're more stressed, your breathing pattern will tend toward a shorter exhalation.

Abdominal breath

This may at first seem like a ridiculously simple exercise, but it's an incredibly good way to create a deep sense of calm and relaxation. It's subtly effective – you really do have to try it to experience its benefits. Relaxed breathing in a semi-supine pose naturally makes your abdomen rise and fall while your chest remains still and relaxed. Providing you can find the space, you can use this technique at any time to alleviate stress. Consciously changing the pattern of your breath to abdominal breathing quickly makes you feel more grounded.

⬥ Lie down with your knees raised and your feet flat. Put a small cushion or yoga block under your head if you wish to. Place your hands on your lower abdomen (over your navel) and let them rest there. Close your eyes and release the back of your body into the floor. Relax your chest totally, and feel the gentle, natural rise and fall of your abdomen beneath your hands as you breathe. Visualize your in-breath as a nourishing, supportive energy filling your abdomen. As you breathe out, imagine stress, pain, anxiety, tension, anger and worry flowing out of your body, leaving you refreshed and relaxed. Breathe like this for as long as it feels good – or at least for 12 breaths.

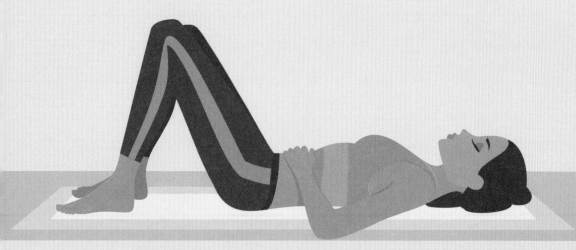

Three-part breath

Generally we all use far less of our breathing capacity than we could. Shallow or restricted patterns of breathing tend to create mental states of anxiety and feelings of being "trapped" or "closed down". The three-part breath is designed to help you to use the whole of your lung capacity at its optimum level, and to calm your body and mind. You can do it while you are sitting, kneeling or lying down. Sitting is perhaps a little more challenging, but you should be well prepared if you've been practising the exercises on the previous pages. If you find this practice uncomfortable, and you feel yourself getting tense around the shoulders, return to one of the practices earlier in this chapter and come back to this one when you feel ready.

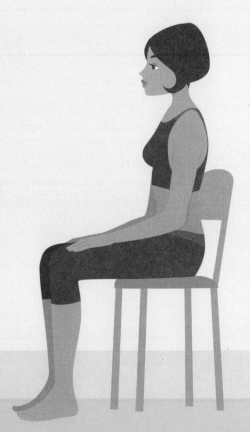 Sit comfortably, with your spine long and effortlessly lifted. Imagine your torso in three sections: base (from the base of your spine to your navel); middle (from your navel to the centre of your chest); and top (from the middle of your chest to the top of your head). Take four breaths into and out of each section in turn, visualizing your breath gently expanding and then relaxing the area. Now try the three-part breath. Inhale into the base section. Pause, and inhale into the middle section. Pause, and then breathe into the top section. Pause for a moment before releasing your breath from all three sections softly and easily. Take a couple of normal breaths, and then repeat this three-part breath six to eight times.

Sitali - mouth breathing

Sitali breath is a wonderful exercise if you feel your temperature rising physically or emotionally. It's said to help cool your body, your mind – and your temper! This is a fantastic practice if you're feeling constantly under pressure, and your moods are swinging toward anger or frustration. It's also one of the very few breathing techniques in yoga that involves breathing in through your mouth.

This breathing technique may help if you suffer from heartburn and indigestion, as it seems to have a cooling and calming effect on the whole stomach area. This area is associated with the element of fire in yoga: although fire is a positive force in the body, it can get a bit out of hand and do damage if you're not careful. You may like to try *sitali* last thing in the evening before you go to sleep, or at any time during the day when you feel irritability or panic start to rise.

⬟ Kneel or sit in a comfortable position. Concentrate on your breathing for a few moments, then roll the sides of your tongue upward to make a tube shape. Stick your tongue out a little bit and lift your chin slightly so your face is tilted upward. Breathe in through the tube created with your tongue. Imagine that you're sipping through a straw. (If you can't roll your tongue, curl the tip of your tongue up until it touches the roof of your mouth – close to your front teeth – and draw in the air around the sides of your tongue.) At the end of your inhalation, gently close your mouth, relax your tongue and let your chin drop down again before you breathe out softly through your nose. Repeat this eight to 12 times.

Humming breath

This is a lovely breathing technique that can relax you and change your mood instantly. According to the theory of yoga, the humming sound itself creates a positive vibration in your body that allows energy to circulate better, freeing accumulated tension and blockages, and resulting in a beautiful, sweet voice. The first time you try it, you may feel slightly silly humming loudly to yourself! After a minute or so you'll get used to the sound, and you can improve its texture, quality and duration quite easily by just listening to the sound you're making. You may be surprised to discover that what you thought was a reasonably steady and full breath sounds a bit feeble when you vocalize it – but don't be discouraged. In a very short time, you can make a huge improvement in the length and quality of your breath.

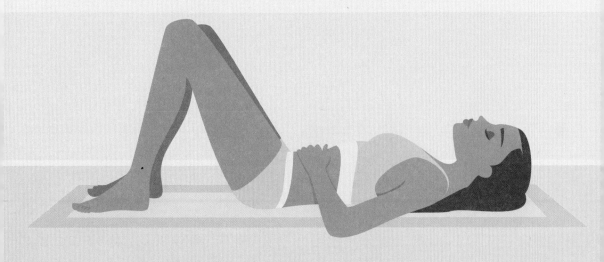

Sit comfortably or lie on the floor with your knees bent and your feet about hip-width apart. Take a few moments to become aware of your breathing, and allow it to settle. Breathe in gently and slowly and then breathe out, making a nice, rounded humming sound.

Continue humming on each out-breath for at least 12 breaths – many more if you feel like it. Experiment with different pitches. The lower ones will resonate in your chest and body; the higher ones in your head and face. Find a pitch that you like and stay with it.

Breath-movement synchronization

This is a wonderful exercise for people who feel tense, tired, agitated or unsettled. It helps to calm your mind and re-centre your attention while effortlessly ensuring that you breathe deeply and for longer. It's an ideal practice for last thing at night, and will aid restful sleep. The movement of your arms is not really a physical exercise, but rather something for your mind and body to follow as you allow your breathing to deepen and develop.

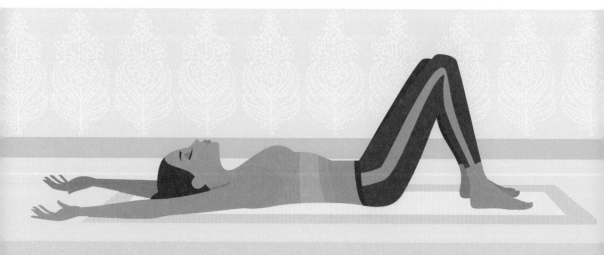

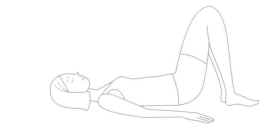

1 Lie on the floor with your knees bent and your feet about hip-width apart. Place a small book, cushion or yoga block under your head if your neck is tense or your chin is tilted up. Rest your arms on the floor by your sides.

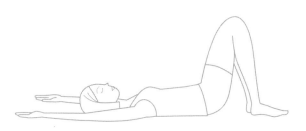

2 As you breathe in, float your arms upward until they touch the floor above your head. See if you can find a position where both your arms are completely relaxed on the floor, and can rest there heavily for a moment. This may mean that you have to bend your elbows or draw your arms out to the sides more – both of these are fine. As you breathe out, gently let your arms float back to the floor beside your hips. See if you can get your movements to synchronize perfectly with your breathing, so that every movement seems to be encapsulated and carried along by your breath.

Repeat steps 1 and 2 eight to 12 times. If you get into a rhythm that you find soothes your mind, keep going for as long as you want to.

Anuloma ujjayi – go with the flow

The Sanskrit term *anuloma* suggests "going with the flow". In this practice you breathe out through one nostril at a time: this makes the out-breath longer, softer and more calming. Because for most people the out-breath is naturally longer than the in-breath, this exercise usually feels fairly easy and natural – hence the name. *Anuloma ujjayi* also helps to balance your body's energetic system.

The hand position you use in this exercise is called *mrgi mudra*, and it consists of curling your index and middle fingers in toward the palm of your hand, leaving your thumb, ring finger and little finger free to close your nostrils. If your arm becomes tired, you can just let it drop back to your lap each time you inhale.

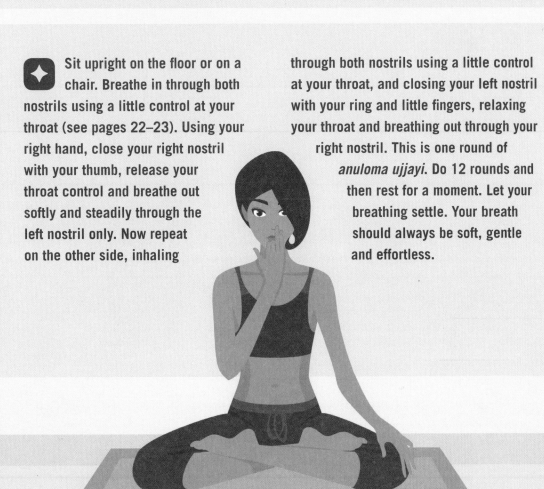

◆ Sit upright on the floor or on a chair. Breathe in through both nostrils using a little control at your throat (see pages 22–23). Using your right hand, close your right nostril with your thumb, release your throat control and breathe out softly and steadily through the left nostril only. Now repeat on the other side, inhaling through both nostrils using a little control at your throat, and closing your left nostril with your ring and little fingers, relaxing your throat and breathing out through your right nostril. This is one round of *anuloma ujjayi*. Do 12 rounds and then rest for a moment. Let your breathing settle. Your breath should always be soft, gentle and effortless.

Daily meditations

Regular meditation can transform your experience of daily life from confusion or agitation to stable, grounded serenity. There are many different meditations and techniques you can try. You just need to find one that feels right for you, and then you'll have the basis of a personal practice you can easily follow.

This chapter contains a variety of simple meditations, ranging from walking meditation, to visualization, to sound meditation. Try all of them, and if you find one that works well, stay with it for a time and see what happens. Used after postures, meditation will deepen and enhance your yoga practice.

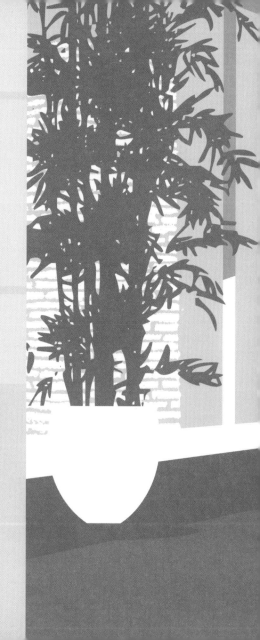

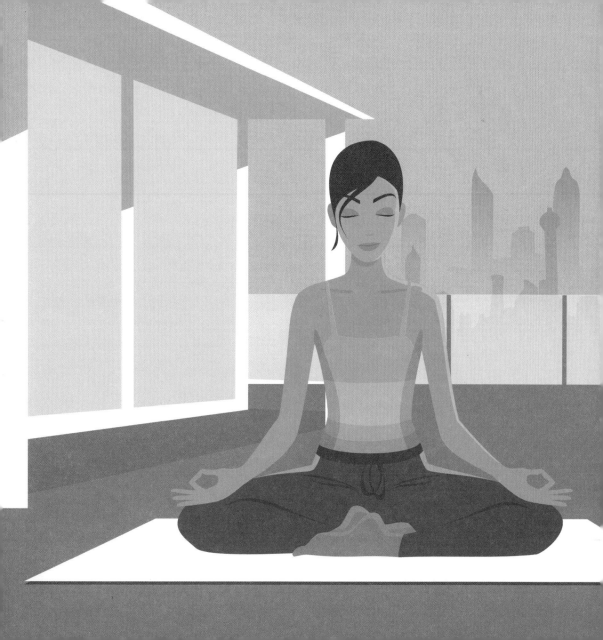

Walking meditation

Although it's most often associated with Buddhism, walking meditation has been used for thousands of years by meditators from a variety of traditions. This kind of meditation is particularly good if, like many people, you find it hard to sit still, perhaps as a result of being physically uncomfortable in a prolonged seated position. Or it may be that the rhythmic and kinetic action of walking helps to soothe and calm your mind, whereas sitting still seems only to agitate it further.

Initially, it's best to practise a walking meditation in an open space where you won't be disturbed. Unless you live in a very grand house, a domestic interior is too small an area in which to do this and you might find yourself pacing about like a caged tiger! Choose a patch of open parkland or garden and, of course, don't do a walking meditation while crossing roads or in other hazardous environments.

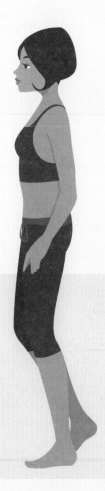 First, just stand still. Notice how your body is balanced, how your feet touch the earth, and how the air feels on your skin. Begin to walk. Your pace should be slow – you're not trying to get anywhere. Be aware of the action of walking. Feel the transfer of weight from foot to foot, and in every step notice the action of your muscles, feet, ankles, knees, hips and torso. Observe the action of your arms too. After a few minutes, stop walking and stand again, maintaining your awareness of your body. Walk again when you feel your awareness drifting. Repeat these walking and still phases for as long as you like.

So hum

In the yoga tradition the sound *so hum* is said to be a spontaneous mantra. It's the sound of the breath, which is with us from the moment of birth to the moment of death. Mantras are special sets of syllables that help us to acheive a meditative state. They're often used like a prayer to encourage positive actions or thoughts, or to release negative ones. You can sing or recite mantras aloud, utter them as whispers under your breath, or repeat them silently (said to be the most powerful way). Mantras are frequently given in initiation rituals, or secretly, by a guru to a disciple. This may make the idea of using a mantra sound a little bit esoteric, but there are some Sanskrit mantras, such as *om* (see pages 122–123) and *so hum*, that have universal appeal – anyone can use them and experience their benefits.

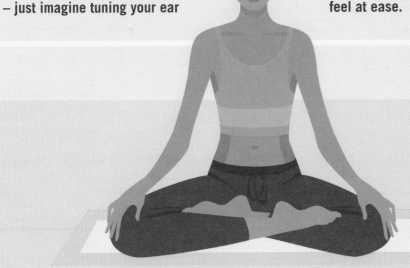

Sit or lie down comfortably. Observe your breath flowing evenly in and out of your body. Let it become fully established at its natural pace. Now imagine that, as you breathe in, you hear the sound "so" and, as you breathe out, you hear the sound "hum". You don't need to make the sounds vocally – just imagine tuning your ear to them. The sound is gentle and soft, but also deep and sonorous, causing a vibration through your body. Stay with the sounds for up to 10 minutes. As you bring your awareness back to everyday life, know that these gentle sounds continue as an undercurrent to your breathing. You can return to them whenever you need to feel at ease.

Chin mudra

This classic hand gesture has almost come to symbolize the practice of yoga. The word *chin* comes from the Sanskrit word for mind, and *mudra* means a seal or lock of energy. *Chin mudra* is often translated as the "seal of consciousness". According to yoga tradition a *mudra* affects the circulation of energy in your body. The name for this energy is *prana*. The seal that you make with your finger and thumb in *chin mudra* creates an energetic circuit of *prana* that helps to develop and sustain higher states of consciousness. You may find that practising *chin mudra* makes you feel more mentally settled, or that it lifts you out of the cycle of thoughts that normally dominates your mind.

You can practise *chin mudra* on its own, or in conjunction with a breathing exercise such as *ujjayi* breath (see pages 22–23), or during meditation. It's a simple hand position that works best if you're seated cross-legged so that your hands can rest on your knees. If this is uncomfortable, practise it sitting in a chair – rest your hands on your thighs. Bring the tips of your index fingers and thumbs together firmly but gently, so they make a ring shape. Allow your free fingers to be open and soft. Let your palms stay open and relaxed, facing upward on your knees. You can hold the *mudra* for as long as you wish, with your eyes open or closed.

Heart *mudra*

Heart *mudra* has a positive influence on your emotions. This *mudra* is said to take the current of *prana* directly to the centre of your chest, which is the seat of an energy centre called *anahata chakra*. According to yoga tradition we gather, store and give out resources of love and compassion from this energy point. In our modern environment, this centre of love can become tight, guarded and shut down by the stresses and strains of daily life. Eventually, this affects not only how we feel emotionally, but it also makes us round-shouldered, hunched or slouched. This in turn impacts on the depth of our breathing and our state of mind. Practising heart *mudra* is an excellent way to keep your heart centre open, vibrant and free!

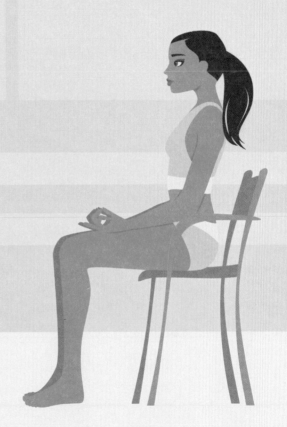 You can practise heart *mudra* anywhere and at any time. You can also combine it with a breathing, meditation or visualization exercise. Rest your hands, palms facing up, on your thighs (or on the floor if you are lying down). On each hand curl your index fingers so that the tips touch the base of your thumbs. Then bring the tips of your ring and middle fingers lightly and firmly to touch the tips of your thumbs. Let your little fingers open out softly away from your palms.

Bring your attention to your heart centre in the middle of your chest. Allow the energy there to open your chest and free your breath. Allow your hands to relax and rest when you feel them tire or start to strain.

Starfish visualization

In this refreshing exercise you imagine your navel as the centre point of your body, and you visualize energy radiating out of it into your feet, hands and the top of your head – these are the five points that form the "starfish". When practising the visualization, it can help to imagine your navel as a point of light or colour, or simply as a place where energy resides. This energy in your core can travel through the whole of your body, nourishing, invigorating and sustaining it, before returning to the navel centre, where it stays as a resource to be called upon when you need it. Watching energy radiating around your body in this way will leave you feeling warm, calm and uplifted – as well as deeply relaxed.

Lie on your back in the resting pose (see pages 86–87), with your feet apart and your arms relaxed and away from your sides, palms facing up. Close your eyes and let your breath settle. Let your body relax heavily into the floor. Imagine energy from your navel centre travelling along your left arm toward your left fingertips. Follow the path of the energy in your mind. Let it return to the navel centre after a couple of breaths. Follow the energy along your left leg to your left foot and back to your navel. Do the same with your right arm and leg. Finally, let the energy move from your navel up to the crown of your head. Imagine it circulating around your head before returning to your navel. Now repeat this "starfish" circuit in the other direction. Return the energy back to your navel centre at the end of the exercise. Give yourself a few moments to let that resource of power stabilize and quieten. Open your eyes, stretch, and sit up slowly.

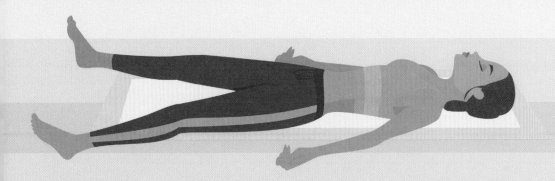

Outer space visualization

This is a simple but highly effective visualization for busy people who feel pressured or consumed by detail or a multitude of tasks. Allowing your mind to escape to a wider perspective for a few minutes can help you regain a sense of proportion when you return to your daily life. If you immerse yourself fully in this visualization, you may find that it takes you a little time to re-acclimatize at the end of the exercise. Rather than jumping up and getting on with your day, treasure this time. Take some deep, steady breaths until you feel ready to return to the day's activities.

Lie on your back in the resting pose (see pages 86–87) and close your eyes. Unless it's very warm, cover yourself with a blanket. Imagine the shape of your body on the floor. Now, in your mind's eye, see the room that you're in; then the building and the street. Imagine an aerial view of the area, then gradually zoom out until you can see the surrounding countryside. "See" the rivers, mountains or valleys, and slowly widen your vision further until you can see the whole continent and the oceans. Keep going until you can see the curve of the Earth and, eventually, the entire planet spinning silently in space. Stay here watching the stars, the Earth and the other planets. Enjoy a sense of weightlessness as you gaze into infinite space. Slowly, like a falling feather, reverse your journey through space until you're back in your own room and body.

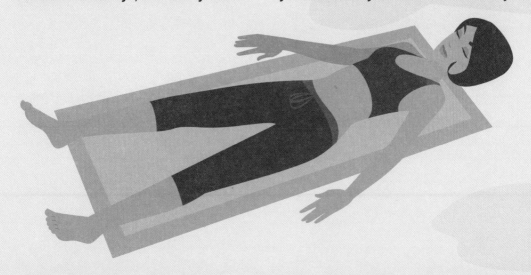

Inner space visualization

Modern life can feel densely packed, with limited personal space and a lot of noise, stimulation and pressure. It's common to feel that we need to "get away from it all" by moving to a place we perceive as more peaceful. But moving home probably isn't practical for most people – and this exercise can make it unecessary! If you turn your mind inward, you may be astonished to discover that your interior space is vast and limitless. And, once you've accessed this space, you may never again feel hemmed in by other people or life's circumstances.

⬥ Lie on your back in the resting pose (see pages 86–87) and close your eyes. Unless it's very warm, cover yourself with a blanket. Observe the weight of your body lying on the floor – make each limb heavy, soft and totally relaxed. Imagine that you weigh five or six times your normal weight. Slowly let your body become light and go on lightening until you are floating. Now return to earth and let your mind relax.

Focus on the space just above and between your eyebrows – visualize a clear blue sky. Imagine that any thoughts that cross your mind are small white clouds. Let them pass across the sky and vanish. There's no need to follow any of your thoughts – just let them drift in and out of the clear blue atmosphere of your mind. Picture this blue sky as limitless, light and open. Remain here as long as you need to fully relax your mind.

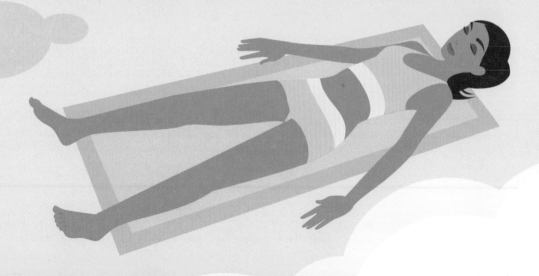

Om

This is the most famous and important of all the mantras in the Indian traditions. It represents the vibration of the universe, and is said to be omnipresent. You can chant it aloud, breathe it quietly, or utter it silently. *Om* is often chanted before and after many other mantras, but you can also use it on its own. *Om* is not translatable into English, as its meanings are so vast, various and undefined – we simply don't have a comparable idea in Western culture.

The Sanskrit symbol for *om* is made up of five parts, which are said to represent the various states of human consciousness. The upper curve represents waking consciousness, the lower one dreaming, the wave moving out to the side stands for deep sleep. The dot represents a transcendental state, and the curve below it the idea of *maya*, or illusion.

✦ Sit in a comfortable position and join your fingers and thumbs in the *chin mudra* (see pages 112–113). To chant *om* aloud, think of it as three separate sounds that are merged: "a", "u" and "m". The humming sound of the "m" at the end should take at least as long as or much longer than the initial vowel sounds. Let your breath settle, then breathe in normally. As you breathe out, chant the sound: "a – u – mmm". Play around with the pitch and tone until the chant sounds right. Over a series of repetitions you'll be able to lengthen your breath and deepen and open the sound into an amazing vibration of your whole body. Do this for as long as you like and, at the end of the last *om*, let the humming sound dissolve into silence. Sit quietly for a moment or two to let your self absorb the "after-*om*" feeling of the sound. This practice has a remarkably soothing and nourishing effect.

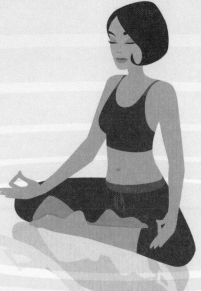

Further reading, CDs and DVDs

If you'd like to learn more about yoga there's a wealth of resources available. Traditionally, yoga is handed down from teacher to student, and this is still the best way to learn if you can find a good local teacher. However, authors and publishers are now producing many excellent books, magazines, CDs and DVDs, and in addition there is a range of wonderful websites, all of which present various aspects of yoga in more detail.

Listed opposite are just a few personal recommendations of tried and trusted materials to get you started. You'll soon get a feel for what interests you and the aspect of yoga that speaks to you most clearly.

BOOKS

Bennett, B. and Greenfield, L. *Emotional Yoga*
(Simon and Schuster, New York, 2002)

Bouanchaud, B. *The Essence of Yoga:*
Reflections on the Yoga Sutra of Patanjali
(Rudra Press, Oregon, 1997)

Desikachar, T.K.V. *The Heart of Yoga*
(Inner Traditions International, New York,
1995)

Farhi, D. *Yoga Mind, Body & Spirit*
(Henry Holt, New York, 2000)

Fraser, T. *Yoga for You*
(Duncan Baird Publishers, London, 2001)

Iyengar, B.K.S. *Light on Yoga*
(HarperCollins, London/New York, 2001)

Satyananda Saraswati *Asana Pranayama*
Mudra Bandha
(Bihar School of Yoga, Bihar, India, 1966)

CDs

Feuerstein, G. *The Lost Teachings of Yoga*
(Sounds True, Boulder, Colorado, 2003)

Freeman, R. *Yoga Matrix*
(Sounds True, Boulder, Colorado, 2003)

DVDs

Desai, G. *Yoga Unveiled*
(Gita Desai, Avon, Connecticut, 2004)

Index

Author's acknowledgments:

Thanks to Zoë Fargher and
Grace Cheetham.